SURVIVING THE PANDEMIC WITH CHILDREN

A Parent's Guide To Living With The New Normal

SANDRA BROWN

TABLE OF CONTENT

INTRODUCTION

Parenting during the corona virus outbreak can put extra weight on families and youngsters. Children are at home full time, many are exploring on the web, school, and parent are telecommuting.

Most guardians would concur this was the most bonkers, disorderly period ever. We were fighting with the dread and change brought about by the corona virus pandemic. Adding to that, we were acclimating to having our children home every minute of every day, isolated inside.

CHAPTER 1

Surviving The Pandemic With Kids

A considerable lot of us were additionally unexpectedly self-teaching our kids. As though that wasn't enough, we were likewise telecommuting, attempting to reconsider childcare, and essentially barely holding on simply attempting to get past every day in one piece.

My principle all through this confused time was, enough should be adequate. If my children endeavored to do their homework, if everybody was taken care of and if my work is completed as well as could be expected that implied that everything was going fine and dandy. Truly, my home was somewhat of a disaster area, we ate solidified meals most evenings, and the children invested an excessive amount of energy in screens. In any case, this wasn't typical life, so I cut every one of us a ton of slack.

How Can We Communicate With Kids About

The Corona Virus?

Indeed, even with little children, you need to be straightforward; however you need to talk at their level. So you probably won't state, "There's COVID-19 – it's making many individuals debilitated and it's causing a great deal of deaths." Clearly, we would prefer not to express that to a 6-year-old, for instance. In any case, you can say: "Individuals are becoming ill as a result of an infection, sort of like this season's cold virus, and we need to ensure that everyone remains sound. Along these lines, we're remaining in our home until further notice and doing school at home."

Young people will clearly have a superior comprehension. They're progressively mindful with the entirety of what's happening. On the off chance that they pose inquiries, help answer those inquiries sincerely as well as could be expected.

Furthermore, in the event that you don't have a clue about the appropriate responses, plunk down together and turn the appropriate responses upward on a believed government site like the Habitats for Infection Control and Counteraction or a trustworthy news site.

What you would prefer not to do is make something up or deceive your young child, since they will discover the other story and afterward they'll be increasingly befuddled.

You need to be straightforward. In any case, it's imperative to assist kids with having a sense of security, keep sound schedules, deal with their conduct and construct flexibility.

Here Are Hints To Help Your Family Through The Pandemic.

Address Your Kids' Anxiety

Kids depend on their folks for security, both physical and emotional. Promise your kids that you are there for them and that your family will get past this together.

Answer Inquiries Concerning The Pandemic Basically And Genuinely

Talk with youngsters about any alarming news they hear. It is alright to state individuals are becoming ill, however state keeping rules like hand washing and remaining at home will enable your family to remain solid.

Recognize Your Kid's Emotions

Gently state, for instance, "I can see that you are vexed on the grounds that you can't have your companions over."

Keep in contact with friends and family

Kids may likewise stress over a grandparent who is living alone or a family member or companion with an expanded danger of getting COVID-19. Video talks can help reduce their tension.

Tell Your Child Before You Go Out For Work Or Basic Tasks

In a quiet and consoling voice, reveal to them where you are going, how long you will be gone, when you will return, and that you are finding a way to remain safe.

Look forward

Reveal to them that researchers are endeavoring to get solutions to help individuals who get sick, and that things will show signs of improvement.

Offer additional embraces and state "I love you" all the more regularly.

Keep solid schedules

During the pandemic, it is a higher priority than any time in recent memory to keep up sleep time and different schedules. They make a feeling of request to the day that offers consolation in an exceptionally dubious time. All kids, including teenagers, enjoy schedules that are unsurprising yet adaptable enough to address singular issues.

Structure The Day

With the standard schedules perplexed, build up new every day plans. Separate homework whenever the situation allows. More seasoned youngsters and teenagers can help with plans, yet they ought to follow an overall request, for example,

- Wake-up schedules, getting dressed, breakfast and some dynamic play during the day, trailed by calm play and to progress into homework.

- Lunch, errands, work out, some online social time with companions, and afterward schoolwork toward the evening.

- Family time and reading before bed.

A Word On Sleep Times

Kids frequently experience more difficulty with sleep time during any distressing period. Attempt to keep ordinary evening time schedules, for example, book, brush and bed for little kids. Put a family picture by their bed for 'additional love' until morning. Sleep times can move for more established kids and youngsters, yet it is a smart thought to keep it in a sensible range so the rest wake cycle isn't perplexed. Too little rest makes it all the more testing to learn and to manage feelings.

CHAPTER 2

Utilize Positive Parenting and Control

Everybody is progressively on edge and stressed during the pandemic. More kids might not have the words to portray their emotions. They're bound to showcase their pressure, nervousness or dread through their conduct (which can, annoy guardians, especially in the event that they are on the edge). More established kids and teenagers might be extra bad tempered as they pass up time with companions and exceptional occasions being dropped.

A few different ways you can enable your kids to deal with their feelings and conduct:

• Redirect awful conduct

Here and there kids get out of hand since they are exhausted or don't have the foggiest idea about any better. Discover something different for them to do.

• Creative play

Recommend your kids to draw pictures of ways your family is remaining safe. Make a composition and hang it up to remind everybody. Or on the other hand, manufacture an indoor stronghold or mansion to keep the germs under control, getting most loved toys or toys.

• Direct your consideration

Consideration - to fortify great practices and dishearten others- - is an incredible asset. Notice great conduct and point it out, applauding achievement and great attempts. Clarifying clear desires, especially with more seasoned youngsters, can help with this.

• **Use rewards and benefits** to strengthen great practices (finishing school tasks, errands and so on.) that wouldn't ordinarily be given during less distressing occasions.

• Know when not to react

For whatever length of time that your kid isn't accomplishing something risky and gets consideration for good conduct, overlooking terrible conduct can be a successful method of halting it.

- **Unique Time In**

Indeed, even with everybody home together day in and day out, put aside some uncommon time with every kid. You pick the time, and let your kids pick the action. Only 10 or 20 minutes of your full attention, regardless of whether just once, will mean a great deal to your kids. Keep mobile phones off or on quiet so you don't get diverted.

• **Avoid physical discipline**

Beating, hitting, and different types of physical or "corporal" discipline causes injury and isn't compelling. Physical discipline can expand hostility in youngsters after some time, neglects to instruct them to act or practice discretion, and can even meddle with typical mental health. Flogging may remove a child's feeling of wellbeing and security at home, which are particularly required at this point.

• Take care of yourself

Parental figures likewise ought to make certain to deal with themselves genuinely: eat healthy, practice and get enough rest. Discover approaches to decompress and take breaks. On the off chance that more than one parent is home, alternate viewing the kids if conceivable.

Remember to calm down

Notwithstanding contacting others for help, guardians feeling overpowered or particularly pushed.

The pandemic has made a significant move in the calendars and ways of life of most families, and it is reasonably adding more pressure and vulnerability to day by day life. Numerous guardians and parental figures have ended up telecommuting while taking on self-teaching their kids.

CHAPTER 3

The New Normal Solution

Here are six hints to help guardians during this "new way of life."

1. Keep Schedule

Keep awakening and hitting the sack simultaneously consistently. Everybody ought to prepare during the day and not hang out in night robe throughout the day. Keep steady supper times.

2. Make a Timetable

Truly work out a noticeable calendar on a bit of paper or white board. This brings a feeling of control and permits you to set desires, which mitigates uneasiness.

You can incorporate significant gatherings you have on this timetable every day, just as assigned. Fix time to play with your children, so they know when they will have exceptional time with you. Take breaks and have lunch or potentially a nibble together.

3. Work When They Rest

It isn't perfect yet attempt to complete work before kids get up during the day, during snooze time and after sleep time. On the off chance that your children despite everything rest, this is likely an advantageous time for telephone calls.

4. Permit More Screen Time

Nonetheless, be clear with your children this is an exceptional time and this won't be a customary event. Setting up virtual play dates through a video stage on an electronic gadget and discovering science/exhibition hall or different exercises online can likewise be useful. Attempt to likewise utilize gadgets to make, for example, drawing or making music.

5. Have Clear Limits

Make a stop light framework for your office space, particularly for more seasoned children. A red light implies that you're occupied, and they can't come in. A green light implies enter! It tells them when they can get to you. Practice this framework ahead of time so everybody is knowledgeable.

6. Incline toward Cooperation (if/whenever the situation allows)

On the off chance that your partner is home, as well, attempt to adjust to and fro who can be accessible for the children. At whatever point conceivable, attempt to part the kid care obligations for the duration of the day and have clear correspondence about when you have significant assembles and conferences.

This will assist everybody with feeling that the basic parts of their day are quiet and without interruption.

Make sure to take it easy on yourself and practice self-care.

CHAPTER 4

Down To Earth Tips For Enduring The

Pandemic

Increased time together in the house can prompt exhausted kids, jumping on one another's nerves, heightening clash, and genuine difficulties to our mental soundness!

Here are some down to earth tips for enduring the pandemic. They are focused at parents of little kids, yet similar standards apply to children of all ages.

1. Split your home

Nothing causes us to lose our marbles speedier than trouble. Family spaces can rapidly slip into horrendous disorganized zones except if an exertion is made to limits various exercises to various zones of the house. Characterize clear zones in your home relating to

1) Adult zone

2) kid play zones

3) Uproarious crude zones;

4) Gentle exercises, etc.

Put a guide of this on the ice chest entryway for all to see.

2. Make a free calendar

Once more, set up a timetable on the refrigerator with arranged exercises to keep your children, and yourself occupied. Make a free timetable for morning, evening and night for every day, multi week ahead of time. Pick a blend of imaginative, learning, and paltry exercises, blended in with ordinary errands for all to partake in. Attempt to make everything as much fun as possible!

3. Plan for remunerations and control

Work out what youngster practices you need to see a greater amount of, what practices you need to see less of, and afterward plan ramifications for both. In this way, positive practices like adhering to guidelines, playing pleasantly, playing freely, and talking pleasantly ought to be compensated with acclaim, nestles, friendship, prizes, and particularly your time.

Battling, hostility, refusal to adhere to guidelines, and other issue practices ought to be met with quiet, clear outcomes like loss of a benefit, or break. The standard here is to ensure you are concentrating on positive kid conduct than negative.

Furthermore, remember, prizes ought to be fun, flighty, enthusiastic, and diverse each time; order ought to be unsurprising, exhausting, and non-passionate.

4. Hold a family meeting

Get together to conceptualize and choose the focuses 1, 2 and 3 above. Include everybody, tune in to your child's sentiments, and keep it fun. "Shake on it" toward the end of the gathering to affirm the family plan (during this emergency, knock elbows!). You need the children to get tied up with the arrangement, so the more they believe they were a piece of the procedure, the better!

5. Give your kid your complete consideration

Plan for committed extraordinary time; say 30 minutes to a great extent every day, for every youngster independently.

6. Focus on your spouse

Plan for devoted parent time and few moments to a great extent, to support yourself and grown-up connections.

7. Try not to engage in battles

Do whatever it takes not to engage in refereeing youngsters' battles. Attempting to discover who began what, and who did what to who isn't valuable and strengthens the battling. Rather, treat the kids as a group, decline to engage in who did what and reward them as a gathering for playing pleasantly, and apply outcomes to them as a gathering, for battling and not playing great.

8. Utilize the Premark standard

A helpful standard in the brain science of learning is that individuals will play out a less preferred undertaking to access a progressively alluring errand. Accordingly, make access to screen time and other profoundly wanted exercises, reliant on having finished errands and schoolwork first!

9. Do a web based child rearing course

Help your youngsters figure out how to act well and be cheerful, by doing a web based child rearing course. This one works! On the off chance that the kids are continually battling, contending, pitching fits and crying and being resistant, with the end goal that you are experiencing difficulty dealing with the kids and your own responses to them, do an online course that shows specific abilities in overseeing issue youngster conduct.

10. Rediscover the love!

At long last, attempt to make this fun and rediscover the adoration. Recollect the positive reasons you needed kids and a family. Discover a spot in your heart for your family and invest as much energy there as possible. Excuse them for minor disturbances, and open up your heart, fraternize, chuckle, and discover love and delight in the easily overlooked details that happen every day and the reality you are together.

CHAPTER 5

Pandemic-Style Summer Ideas

There really are a ton of fun things children can do this mid-year, while remaining safe. As it were, this may be one of the most vital summers for families around the globe and possibly yours as well.

Here are my top suggestions:

1. Patio fun

Not every person has a patio we in reality just have a yard we share with others in our high rise. On the off chance that you have no outside territory to call your own, you can go to a recreation center during "off hours" and locate an uninhabited zone to call your own. Most children are only glad to play openly outside, yet on the off chance that you need somewhat more structure, have a go at sorting out a straightforward fortune chase or make an impediment course for your children.

2. Climbing

Climbing is extraordinary on the grounds that there are typically approaches to remain securely removed from others. Additionally, prepare in the event that you are taking children on the grounds that, contingent upon their age, they can tire rapidly. Pick a basic climb with adequate spots to rest.

Outdoors

Outdoors is a superb method to travel during a pandemic in particular because of the outside and the capacity to socially distance properly. Getting ready to camp can be a great deal of work for guardians, yet outdoors can be a fun and paramount experience for the little ones.

Virtual day camp

Numerous camps are going on the web this late spring, and keeping in mind that you and your children might be worn out from web based learning, day camps are about fun and innovative exercises. Many are offering virtual workmanship, sports, and move exercises.

Virtual and socially distanced play dates

On the off chance that your kid is mature enough to adhere to social removing rules, having a play date with a family who is in the same spot about security rules can be a pleasant break. Meeting outside in a zone that considers appropriate distancing, not sharing things like tidbits and beverages, and trying to keep those covers on, are your most secure wagers.

Water play

In the event that you have a terrace, this is the ideal opportunity to get a good old inflatable pool. In the event that you don't have your own space, you can whip out some water inflatables, or water squinters. So fun! Sea shores and lakes might be open in your general vicinity, as well. Discover when the "off-hours" are to stay away from groups and avoid potential risk.

Drive-in motion pictures

Numerous towns are equipping with this retro legacy and setting up drive-in motion pictures. Bring cushions and snacks, and appreciate. I can hardly wait to give this a shot with my family. I haven't been to a drive-in since I was a little child.

While we will be unable to return to cinemas for some time, summer is the ideal chance to appreciate open air motion pictures with your family.

As a last resort, let them be exhausted

This maybe the most significant suggestion I can give you (and I have to hear it as well). You don't need to engage your children each second of the mid-year break.

A large number of us will in any case be working while our children are home. There will be numerous hours where they cry about how exhausted they are. Be that as it may, fatigue is really something worth being thankful for. If you let your child sit with their weariness for some time that is frequently when the best time, innovative play develops.

Thus, let them be exhausted. The greater part of our children are overscheduled and over invigorated for what it's worth. A late spring of nothing may, over the long haul, be useful for their spirits. What's more, when in doubt, you can let them daydream for a couple of hours before the television or a computer game. All things considered, it's everything about equalization.

CHAPTER 6

How To Help Your Child Intellectual And

Psychological Wellbeing

School's out

As schools all over the world stops to curb the spread of corona virus, a huge number of kids are obliged to stay at home. You don't need them accomplishing their work on their bed or simply relaxing on their bed with the PC doing their homework. You truly need to have them at a table or a work area, a region that is assigned for their homework so you're keeping those spaces depicted. Just as keeping your kid on an ordinary calendar, similar to you would during the school week. Sleep time ought to be the equivalent, getting them up simultaneously during the day.

Being extremely aware of those spaces for your kids and checking in with them to ensure they aren't getting dismal nor have stresses and questions. Great deals of the adolescents that I've worked with are really doing very well with this situation. They're modifying likely better than their folks are.

During this time, it is useful for guardians to think about their kid's requirements for structure, work out, social contact, fitting relaxation time and quiet, sane clarifications about the circumstance.

A Requirement for Structure

Kids may believe this opportunity to be like long school breaks or summer get-away, however it isn't actually the equivalent. Not at all like summer get-away, this break is abrupt and spontaneous, and the time away from school has not been indicated. This can be hard for kids to understand. All in all, individuals don't do well when they are uncertain about the future, even in a zone as straightforward as the calendar.

Set a calendar for the weekdays and ends of the week. Kids and youngsters give a valiant effort if there are plans for every day, particularly the weekdays when they would have been in school.

Set Standard Sleep times and Wake-Ups

After maybe the initial days, have your kid follow the standard school day–end of the week day rest plan. It is ideal to have a normal wake-up time and sleep time that is equivalent to the timetable you set when they are going to class, since it tends to be difficult to refocus, particularly if kids get into a late-to-bed, late-to-rise plan.

Build up a School Day Instructive Timetable

In an out of control situation, free timetable is pleasant for snow days or other brief breaks, yet can prompt weariness and a troublesome time getting once again into the instructive daily schedule in the event that it keeps going. Discover how your kids' schools intend to keep students connected with and follow the recommended plan.

Guardians can consider beginning with an early daytime meeting and timetable rundown, since this is the thing that most educators do to begin the day. Have a rundown of the subjects and exercises for the afternoon, and make 30-to 45-minute squares of time to take a shot at the subjects that your youngster takes.

For younger grade students, a good example of morning could incorporate math, trailed by a mobile break or playing for around 10 minutes; social investigations—including recent developments—used on the web assets; a lot of bouncing jacks and a race around the house for another break; and afterward science.

Taking Training on the Web

While schools are covered, numerous schools are moving their exercises online by giving virtual guidance or tasks. Ensure your kid stays aware of the tasks and can take part in any virtual guidance.

In the event that your kid's school isn't giving these alternatives, divert to sources from legitimate self-teach associations and sites, the same number of these associations give exercises and materials to each review level.

Exercise and Social Contact

By doing exercises every day, everybody will be more settled and will rest better. Get included by going for strolls and messing around with your children, for example, tag, find the stowaway, Red Wanderer. Transfer races, bicycle rides, and climbs are extraordinary, as well. Climbs can likewise be utilized to educate about nature, plants, creatures, and fowls.

Concerning sports, you can get all together of children to play a few games. It doesn't need to be extravagant—kickball is appreciated by all ages.

Follow rules on the sheltered size of gathering contacts that individuals can have, depending on the CDC or your neighborhood office of general wellbeing for direction. Getting companions together in little gatherings can give fun and straightforwardness strain. Social contact is significant for kids. Youth that are associated with other youngsters are more joyful, less restless, and have a great time.

In any event, when secluded, guardians can assist kids remain associated with others with current innovation, inside sensible cut-off points. Empower suitable and sensible utilization of telephones, tablets, and PCs for making the associations. Guardians ought to follow shrewd direction on use, including expansive checking of substance and the tone of interchanges that have been or are happening.

You don't have to know the subtleties of every communication, except you ought to have a feeling of the subjects and the people that your youngster is reaching, even adolescents. While out of school, youngsters might be viewed as expected focuses for digital predators, so urge your kids to be open about the messages that they get and people that are reaching endeavors.

Relaxation Time and Meditation

Let your children have a differed recreation time diet of TV, books, and other media. A portion of the substance can be serious and elevating, and a littler segment of it very well may be senseless or even junky.

Verify that a decent segment of relaxation time action is dynamic, both intellectually and materially. Inactive perception and watching of shows is fine, however don't release your kid's psyche numb by devouring substance that doesn't require thought. Instructors and school give kids over six hours of mental exercise. Attempt to coordinate that.

Inactive and stationary amusement can likewise be an issue. It can prompt a decrease in physical wellbeing and wellness and add to undesirable weight gain. Keep in mind, at school; kids are at any rate strolling around the structure.

Diminishing Nervousness Even with Genuine Concerns

It's best for guardians to give judicious clarifications about COVID-19 and help keep up a fitting quiet, specialist's state. To help oversee tension in offspring everything being equal, make sure to give precise data from solid sources.

Perceive that even little youngsters catch discussions and news reports. Kids state that they discover nearby news that they don't comprehend to be more terrifying than startling fantasies or even blood and gore films. Along these lines, it's significant for guardians to ask their children on the off chance if they have inquiries or worries about the circumstance and to make a solid effort to explain their understandings.

Put forth a valiant effort to shield your kids and relatives from COVID-19 and let your kid know how they can secure themselves as well as other people. Aides and rules for social distancing and cleanliness and talking with medicinal services experts ought to be followed. Indeed, even little youngsters can smoothly get sicknesses.

Tell them at a fitting formative level how COVID-19 can be passed onto others, which many people don't turn out to be debilitated, and that wellbeing experts are endeavoring to deal with the virus in detached settings.

If you are relaxed, unreasonably stressed, tense, or miserable, talk with wellbeing, psychological well-being, and different wellsprings of directing, for example, church. Check for these responses in your kids as well. Unpleasant occasions add to psychological wellness issues, particularly in the event that they were available before the pressure begun.

Try to deal with you and your kids' psychological well-being during this health concern. Take part in sensible interruptions and have your kids do likewise. Consider checking the news once in a while instead of checking it continually.